THE ZERO EFFORT DIET

DRINK BEER
EAT JUNK
GET FIT

Copyright © Nick Baynes
ALL RIGHTS RESERVED

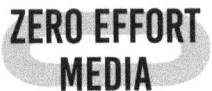

ZERO EFFORT
MEDIA

ISBN-13: 978-1512060775
ISBN-10: 1512060771

CONTENTS

INTRODUCTION

Whether you're looking to lose weight, tone up, or simply stay in shape, choosing the right approach can be hard. Almost every diet or exercise plan out there requires you to stick religiously to their precise set of rules. Watch your calories. Cut down on fat. No, actually, cut out sugar. Don't do that, have no gluten instead. Don't count calories. Eat more meat! Cut out meat. Only eat normally for three days a week. Fast! Don't fast! And on, and on, and on…

There's rarely a suggestion that you can pick and choose from whichever approach you want (no doubt partly because many of these fitness gurus are also peddling supplements, or website subscriptions, so want to lock you into their routine exclusively).

In this day and age we've been taught that you don't need to be locked into just one thing that's presented to you. We no longer buy albums, we make playlists of our favourite songs on Spotify. We don't require a TV network to tell us when we can watch our favourite shows, we watch on demand, when and where we want. Even in politics the concept of all or nothing is changing, as coalitions and minority governments around the world become more common.

So why does choosing the right healthy lifestyle feel like something you have to sign up to exclusively?

Not only that, almost every program out there involves eliminating *something* from your diet. This leads to binge dieting, yo-yoing on and off, seeing fast gains before willpower is broken and you double down back on your old unhealthy lifestyle.

This book cuts through the crap and presents the best tips and habits to adopt from a wide variety of approaches. All either involve minimal willpower, or eliminating nothing from your diet (unless you want to), and encourage you to enjoy your life while being healthy. Rather than suggesting you follow all of them, or stick to solely these choices, this book encourages you to pick a couple at a time, try them, see what works, and then try some others.

If you're looking for a plan to take you to professional athlete levels of fitness or to get a body like a pro bodybuilder, then this won't help you (initially). For the rest of us though, just trying a few of these tips at a time will see genuine changes to your body, your energy levels, and your overall wellbeing.

Why listen to me?
I'm not a doctor or a personal trainer, or in fact sporty in any way. My job involves sitting in front of a computer screen all day, and going to conferences where drinking and eating to excess are the norm.

From being a scrawny teenager, I became an overweight 20-something. By thirty I was nudging 17 stone on the scales, with a double chin and worse acne than when I was a teenager. Shortly after that my bathroom scales and mirror finally convinced me that something had to be done. What followed was a decade of trying one diet after another, a variety of different training routines, and massive weight loss followed by massive weight gains.

A couple of years ago, I realised that I'd acquired enough knowledge that I should just start following what I knew actually worked for me, wherever the original inspiration came from. The result was that without cutting back on my social life, continuing to drink beer and eat junk once or twice a week, I rapidly hit my target weight and body shape. By the time I'd hit 40 I was over four stone lighter than when I was a decade younger, losing weight in a steady and consistent fashion, and had energy levels peak back to how they were twenty years previous.

This book contains many of the tricks and tips I've followed in that journey. I'm not suggesting you try all of them at once. If you do you're likely to give up as it will be just another fad lifestyle change. I'd recommend reading through them all, then picking out two or three that sound best for you. If they work, then that's great - now add a couple more at your own pace. If you've found that the ones you first tried didn't work for you, drop them and try some more.

Not only should you see and feel tangible changes, as you won't have given up anything you should be able to stick to it. That's then a great platform to take things to the next level (if you choose to). I've recently switched to a plant only diet as an experiment, and it's working great for me. I could never have jumped straight into that without doing everything in this book first though. If and when I drop this diet then I know that as long as I stick to the rules in these pages I'll be OK.

This book is structured in a way that is short, to the point, and with no BS. First of all we'll discuss tips regarding your diet before moving onto a section focusing on fitness. There's a short chapter on ways to minimise damage when you have a really big night out or weekend, before a final chapter covering various resources that help with all the tips throughout.

I hope you find the Zero Effort Diet life changing. I wish I'd had it ten years ago before I'd spent weeks and months bouncing from one extreme diet to another!

Let me know your progress at nick@nickbaynes.com and sign up to my newsletter at www.tinyurl.com/zero-effort to receive more content for free every month.

Nick Baynes

DIET

The Zero Effort Diet

1. The Low Fat Myth

So let's get this one out of the way first. If you just go into a supermarket and browse the healthy aisles you'll be bombarded with items that are screaming "low" and "reduced" fat, implying that if you buy them it will be the first step towards becoming a healthier you.

The simple advice here is, don't fall for it! Firstly, by reducing the fat the manufacturers will have normally compensated with something else, normally more salt or sugar. Technically you're reducing your fat intake but increasing how much other "bad" stuff you're eating (see "Low Sugar" and "Reduced Salt" packaging for the same tactics).

The next thing to bear in mind is that while it may contain lower fat than the regular version of the product, it doesn't mean it's actually "low" in fat. Yes you'll be consuming less fat than the regular version, but no, it doesn't guarantee that you're suddenly eating a low fat diet.

The final and most important reason to forget about the low fat myth, is that generally if you follow just a few of the other tips in this guide then you don't really need to worry about fat content anyway. Fat is needed by the body, it's the saturated fat which is the bad stuff. If you're a bit more active and follow just a few of the guidelines in this book, then that should cancel out the need to worry about your intake.

Psychologically (which is an underrated factor in staying in shape) you're going to feel a lot better about yourself, because you won't be buying food that your brain is telling you is going to taste worse than your regular items. If you want to buy some sausages for example, and you normally buy the regular, full fat, varieties, then go ahead and carry on. As long as you're following some of the other tips here you'll still lose weight and feel good.

2. How to Beat Your Sweet Tooth

When I was growing up, until I was around 17, I didn't really have much of a sweet tooth. I liked bitter dark chocolate but my snacks of choice were definitely savoury. When I was diagnosed with Type 1 Diabetes that all changed. I began to associate sugary junk (chocolate, jelly beans, Skittles, energy drinks, etc.) with the sweet sugary nectar that would save my life if I had low blood sugar.

As a result, I found that I didn't just develop a sweet tooth, but a whole mouthful of them.

Obviously for me as a diabetic that's not good, but for regular people that's not great either. Eating sugary, simple carbs, sends your sugar levels soaring, followed by the inevitable crash later on (at which point you have two choices, feel like crap, or eat more chocolate. I know which I choose).

Also, ironically, you get a double whammy of fat forming issues with this scenario as your body produces insulin to bring the blood sugar levels back down - and increased insulin in your body increases your body's fat storage potential.

In the spirit of getting healthy without giving anything up then, how do we conquer the sweet tooth problem? One simple word - Cacao.

Cacao beans are the main ingredient that chocolate is made from. Go to your local health store and buy a pack of powdered cacao, open it up and breath in that amazing chocolatey smell (buy it first). Because it's pure, unsweetened, powdered cacao beans the nutritional information is incredibly healthy - per 100 grams, around 1.5 grams sugar (and around 27 grams of natural protein, which we'll come to later).

Sounds too good to be true, and in a way it is. Stick a teaspoon of the powder in your mouth and that sweet chocolatey smell soon turns into a bitter, mouth drying gag. This is where sweetener comes in. I use Truvia (made from the leaves of the stevia plant) but any sweetener will do (apart from sugar, duh!).

With these two ingredients, the world is your oyster. If you love coffee then mix in a half a teaspoonful of cacao with your sweetener, for a mochaccino style drink without any of the sugar. Mix cacao powder with cacao butter, add some sweetener, and put in the freezer to set, and you have sugar free, high protein, healthy chocolate. As you're saving sugar and fat content in the chocolate if you want to put other regular candy treats into the mix then go for it. You'll still have a healthy chocolate bar compared to regular treats from super market.

(A note on Truvia - this sugar free sweetener is my personal favourite as it smells of candy floss when you open the pack. My brain gets the happy chemicals associated with eating pure sugar without even putting anything in my mouth).

If I really still have a craving then I find playing Candy Crush on my phone tricks my brain into thinking my sweet tooth is being satisfied too. Sadly, I'm being serious.

3. Control Chips and Go Nuts

I know I just said I have a sweet tooth but give me a family size bag of tortilla chips and I'll happily eat my way to the bottom before I've realised it.

With sugar our bodies have a natural cut off that tells us we've eaten too much, but unfortunately we don't know how to stop eating fatty savoury snacks. If we switch our consciousness off, then our body won't automatically tell us to stop, even though it should be screaming in our faces "WHAT ARE YOU DOING?!!". We have no inbuilt off switch for fat.

Unfortunately, this means we have to rely on willpower, which isn't easy when everything tastes this good.

There's no silver bullet solution, but here are a few tips that mean you don't have to banish savoury treats from your larder -

- Leave the bag in the kitchen. Don't take it back to the couch, or back to your computer desk, with you. Pour a small amount into a bowl, and take that with you instead. You're far less likely to keep eating if you have to keep getting out of your seat to eat more

- Grab a drink when you grab the snack (ideally not sugary soda!). Try and have a full glass of water or squash when you're eating. This will fill you up more quickly, and make it even less likely you're going to be heading back for another portion.

- Stock up on gum. If you stick some minty chewing gum in your mouth after you've eaten, you're not going to carry on eating after that first bowl. Minty Doritos? No thanks.

- If you like nuts, then try and get them in your larder instead of fried potato and corn snacks. Even though they're still not good for you in excess, in smaller servings they actually have some good fats and protein compared to the empty calories in the other snacks.

Of course, as with many of these tips, if you're able to completely eliminate potato crisps from your diet then you'll reap the benefits. However, if you completely abstain then it's likely your body will crave them more and more, so it's far better to try the above and eat them in moderation than to cut them out and then get back to bingeing within a couple of weeks.

4. Make Your Own Junk

Maybe your willpower is great. Maybe you've made many small changes to your diet and lifestyle and are living a healthier existence than in the past. None of this matters when you walk past a Burger King, or McDonalds, or KFC, and get a whiff of those smells being pumped out through the open doors.

Unless you've never enjoyed fast food, those aromas will go right up your nostrils and hit the button marked "I need some NOW" in your brain.

(Writing this, I'm realising how important smell is to avoiding temptation. Maybe someone should make some diet-friendly nose plugs?)

The good news is that if you're only giving in to those smells once or twice a month then it won't affect your healthy living at all, so go in and indulge yourself!

If you want to stay on top of these cravings though, making your own junk food at home is a great solution. Buy a lean steak burger from your local butchers, grab a load of salad, and get a multigrain roll. Stick it all together with some ketchup and mustard, along with some homemade potato wedges, and you have an enormous, filling, but healthy burger and fries replacement.

Online there are hundreds of resources to be found showing you how to recreate fast food junk with healthy fresh ingredients at home (for example, a five second Google search threw up this recipe for how to make a DIY healthy Big Mac - http://www.cinnamonspiceandeverythingnice.com/homemade-big-macs/).

This won't stop you being tempted when you walk past the fast food joints in the street, but it will add a few layers of cast iron willpower to help you stop walking in.

5. Secret Weapon #1 - Boiled Eggs

If you don't like eggs, or you're following a vegan diet, then this secret weapon is a dud, I'm sorry.

For everyone else - this will transform your daily cravings and food intake.

Here's how the boiled egg secret weapon works.

- identify when you are normally most hungry and susceptible to snacking (normally mid-morning / late afternoon for most people)

- get two pre-boiled eggs out of your bag

- eat them

Sprinkle a little salt on top of them if you want, and enjoy every mouthful of both eggs. Not only will your hunger dissipate, but also your energy levels will rise and you'll find you'll make it through to the next mealtime with ease.

Eggs are high in protein which tells your body that you're full up and will satiate your hunger for at least a couple of hours. People used to be worried about the cholesterol levels of eggs but it's now commonly accepted that eggs contain the good type of cholesterol so popping a couple a day won't do you any harm.

The only thing which may do you harm is your co-workers and friends when you crack them open. If you can find some pre-boiled eggs in your local supermarket or online, then this minimises that smell problem considerably. If not, it might be best to step outside for an egg break...

6. To Dairy or not to Dairy

A number of health plans recommend that you eliminate dairy completely from your diet. It's something I've tried and I've found that when it's cut out that I feel less bloated, and tend to maintain/lose weight more easily.

The big caveat here is that I have never been a big consumer of dairy products. Other than cheese, and having milk in my coffee (and over the years I've managed to acquire a taste for black) dropping it hasn't been hard. I can see that if you have milk with your cereal and drink copious amounts of tea during the day it might be harder for you than me.

Soya milk is actually pretty drinkable (reduced sugar if possible). Many years ago I tried rice milk – which I now avoid at all costs, it put me off non-dairy for a decade!

If you love your milk I wouldn't worry too much about cutting it out. It might be worth trying to see how you go, but if dropping it makes you feel depressed about skipping the cheese aisle, and turns your tea and coffee habits into a chore, then not giving it up won't make a massive difference.

If you're trying to get truly ripped and are aiming for an athlete's body, then removing dairy products is definitely something to consider. For the rest of us though, don't feel like you're letting yourself down by ignoring various dietary advice out there. Just make sure you're making improvements to your food intake elsewhere.

7. Fruit - Chew, Don't Gulp

For a long time I cut fruit entirely out of my diet, mainly due to how high in (natural) sugars they are. I figured that as long as I was getting my vitamins elsewhere it wasn't worth the sugar and insulin spikes.

After reading a lot of different articles about fruit and the benefits, I've revised my thinking. The mantra I now live by when it comes to fruit is "Chew, Don't Gup".

If you **eat** fresh fruit then you're getting the vitamins and goodness, plus the fibre content. There's a high sugar content but it's one portions worth. It's easy to keep to one item of fruit per portion, so you know how much you're eating. Eating fruit in this way avoids those sugar/energy spikes, and is how they were intended to be eaten when hanging off the tree or bush.

Smoothies and fruit juices on the other hand, lose a lot of the fibre content, and contain the sugars from multiple fruits. Look at the nutritional details of store bought smoothies - you may as well be glugging a vitamin tablet with a can of non-diet cola. In one drink that can be gulped down in seconds you're taking in the sugars from multiple portions of fruit. As it's liquid, your body will be tricked into thinking it's less filling than eating something that it still has to break down and digest. Even if you're juicing your own fruit drink at home you're losing the benefits of eating it whole.

The rule then, is that if you have to **chew** it, then that's good for you. Eat fruit and make it part of your daily snack routine.

If you're **drinking** it, then you're losing a lot of the benefits, and guzzling huge amounts of sugar.

Remember, "Chew, Don't Gulp".

8. Vitamin Supplements

The truth is if you're eating a balanced diet then you don't really need vitamin supplements. Having said that as an insurance policy, taking a top up of some of the vital vitamins every morning is no bad thing.

However, don't waste your money on vitamin tablets. The body finds it hard to digest the cases that they come in, and depending on what else you've eaten, much of the good stuff inside just ends up coming out the other end. The result is a highly nutritious shit in your toilet bowl, but that's not really what we're going for (we've all heard of people drinking their own urine for the health benefits, but... urgh, let's not even go there).

The best way of getting those extra vitamins is through effervescent tablets. The big branded tablets can be expensive, but most supermarkets do their own versions, with identical contents, for at least half, if not a quarter of the price.

The other great benefit of effervescent tablet vitamin drinks, is that they can replace your morning glass of orange juice - which is handy given the concept of "Chew, Don't Gulp".

9. Buying Meat - Avoiding the "Con" in Convenience

Don't waste your money on meat from the supermarket. While their practises are improving, many add water to their chicken, do cuts of beef that are overly generous with the fat, and buy their produce from mass produced farms (or rather, factories) where diets and conditions aren't great.

If you go to your local butchers, or farmers market, or an online specialist and shop around, you can get much bigger, leaner, and healthier cuts for your money. Honestly, comparing chicken breast sizes to those bought from smaller suppliers is incredible. Here in the UK I use an online company called Musclefood.com for all my meat purchases. They're cheaper than the supermarkets, and better in every way I just described.

(If you go to their website with this special link, you'll get four chicken breasts for free - http://www.musclefood.com/NB18814)

Whether you buy meat online, from a butchers or a farmers market, I'd recommend avoiding the big chains where possible unless it's your only choice. This tip helps your wallet as well as your waist, so that's this book paid for already with just one bit of advice.

10. Secret Weapon #2 - Lemon Water

Squeeze a lemon into a glass of water twice a day (half a lemon in the morning, the other half in the afternoon), and prepare to be amazed. This is such a simple trick that will turbo charge all of your other health goals.

The water itself will taste a little bitter, which if you like lemons isn't a problem, as it just tastes, well, lemon-y. If you're not a fan still try and drink this as the benefits are worth it.

- Lemon water contains pectin fibre, which helps fight hunger cravings (drink this then have your boiled eggs and wave goodbye to feeling hungry).

- It cleanses your system - lemon juice helps energise your liver enzymes and provides a daily "detox"

- Gives you a natural vitamin C boost (and potassium, calcium, phosphorus, magnesium). Lemons actually have a higher density of vitamin C than oranges.

- Some people believe lemons hold diuretic-like properties. In other words, something that helps your body naturally release some of the water weight it's holding onto. They're not officially included in lists of diuretics but there's no denying that drinking lemon water every day is a big booster when it comes to weight loss.

Try it for a week - you'll notice the difference.

11. Drink Beer and Get Away With It

Now we're onto the important stuff. Beer is mainly water, and made from natural ingredients, so drink as much of it as you can, as often as you can.

Ah. OK. I'm joking.

You probably shouldn't drink it all the time and as much as you want, if you're trying to stay healthy.

However, the good news is that once a week you can pretty much do what you want. As long as you're trying to be healthy the rest of the time it won't make much difference to your progress (it will slow things down, but that's it).

In fact as long as we're talking drinking in moderation, a couple of additional times during the week isn't going to affect things too much either. Remember, the idea behind this book is to keep fit while enjoying life.

- Red wine every day is fine. If you limit yourself to a glass or two of red (Cabernet Sauvignon and Merlot in particular) then you'll notice practically no difference to your weight and progress. If you're the type of person who likes a drink at home in the evening to unwind, try and go with the red wine.

- Some people recommend having a glass of water in between every pint of lager. I can only assume these people have never actually drunk in a pub before. Like that's ever going to happen. A better approach is to try and switch from pints to bottles. Over the course of a couple of rounds you'll be drinking a lot less, but won't feel like you're missing out.

- When you do go out and drink too much don't give up and feel like you've let yourself down. Just move on and carry on with your regular healthy diet. Even if you've drunk to excess, if you had fun, consider it a positive sign that you're comfortable with mixing hedonism with healthy living (note: don't do this every night.)

- Eat before drinking. It's hard to do this sometimes but if you can it will help avoid that feeling of hunger later in the night (when thanks to alcohol you'll be craving everything BUT the healthy options), and it helps absorb and slow down your drinking. Eating ain't cheating.

- If you live in England, leave the UK. Our drinking culture here immediately puts us at a disadvantage to other more sensible nations. Hic.

12. The Most Important Meal of the Day

Your Mum was right, breakfast really is the most important meal. Skip it, or eat something unhealthy, and your energy levels will jump on a rollercoaster for the rest of the day.

As busy adults with work and school runs and a million other things to do in the morning, it's hard to eat right. Ideally you want something that's high in protein, and with a low glycaemic index, meaning that the energy will be released slowly throughout the morning. Not easy to rustle up when you've overslept and need to run out of the door ASAP.

The best thing to do to make sure you're always eating a breakfast that meets nutritional goals is to have something pre-prepared that removes the need to make anything in the morning.

As a backup I try to always have some multi-grain breakfast bars in my larder. They're not as nice or filling as a fresh breakfast, but for convenience they can't be beaten (you can even eat them walking down the road if you really need to). Just make sure you check they're genuinely nutritionally balanced and not actually sugar laden candy bars in disguise. Look for words like "wholegrain", "slow release" and "high in fibre" on the packaging to assist.

My breakfast of choice is chocolate-banana overnight oats. These are made with cacao, sweetener, banana, water, and soya milk (regular milk works too). Mix two tablespoons of cacao, two of sweetener, and a banana together in a bowl. Add half a cup of rolled oats, and one and a half cups of soya milk. Pour into two bowls and leave overnight.

The result in the morning is the freshest, healthiest, tastiest and chocolatey-ist breakfast you can imagine. It keeps for a couple of days so I get two breakfasts out of every batch. I sprinkle fresh blueberries on top of mine, but you don't need to. Delicious.

If that doesn't sound like your type of thing look around online and try and find something you can pre-prepare with a similar nutritional breakdown. Your goal is to avoid those hunger pangs before lunch, and a good breakfast is the foundation behind all of your health goals.

(If you've over indulged the night before then having a ready-made breakfast also helps resist the temptation of going with something fried instead. The benefits of preparation for the morning really can't overstated)

Banana Chocolate Chia Overnight Oats
2 tbsp. Water
2 tbsp. Truvia
1 small Banana
2 tbsp. Cacao Powder
1 cup rolled Oats
3 tbsp. Chia Seeds
1.5 cups Light Soya Milk

Mix water, sweetener, cacao and banana together in a bowl.

Add chia seeds and rolled oats and mix in.

Pour soya milk into bowl while stirring for even consistency.

Split over two breakfast bowls and store in the fridge overnight.

Indulge yourself with fresh berries sprinkled on top in the morning!

13. The Best Dinner Ever

I can't tell you what your best dinner ever is, but I can tell you mine – Inferno Chilli.

- One onion, one red pepper, four mushrooms, one clove of garlic, all finely chopped.
- 400 grams of extra lean minced beef.
- Two Scotch Bonnet Chillies
- 1 teaspoon of hot chilli powder
- One tin of mixed beans
- Two cups of Tomato Passata

Brown the mince in a large pan, add the other ingredients. Leave to simmer for 10 minutes. Pour half in a container for tomorrow and when cooled put in the fridge. Smother the other half with black pepper and dried chilli flakes, and eat (and cry a little at the heat).

This is my best dinner ever for two reasons.

Firstly, it tastes amazing, and I never get bored of the explosion of flavours in my mouth. Secondly, it's easy to make, and is enough for two days. Just like breakfast if I have something easy to make, or already prepared, the temptation for eating junk is almost entirely removed.

Find out what your best dinner ever is and eat it again, and again, and again.

If you get bored of it, find an even better one. Remove the thought process of what to eat and suddenly sticking to your diets becomes a lot easier.

14. Secret Weapon #3 - Sugar Free Jelly

Sweet desserts are a great palate cleanser. Having polished off a big meal, whether healthy or otherwise, wrapping it up with something sweet and indulgent is something that a great many of us have been brought up expecting as part of our dinner time routine.

Unfortunately, ice cream, tiramisu, cheesecake, even some yogurts, are high in sugar, and to a lesser degree salt and fat, so if you're looking for an easy win to reduce a large part of your daily "bad" intake, dessert is often where it's tempting to start.

This of course means that every single mealtime you're reminding yourself that you've given something up. A fast track to failure.

I've found that having a small pot of sugar free jelly is a great way to fool my brain into thinking I haven't really restricted my diet from anything.

Different brands vary, but the sugar free variants are often less than 10 calories, with practically no sugar, salt or fat, yet taste fruity and tangy beyond those values. My brain is obviously a bit stupid, as I know it's just a small pot of jelly and nothing indulgent, but eating that jelly fills the dessert hole, and doesn't leave me craving more. Another great, simple and cheap secret weapon to have in your arsenal.

15. Eat more Plants

Recently I've been eating an exclusively plant based diet (effectively a vegan diet but without the political views or sandals). As a diet it's been incredible, with rapid weight loss and my energy levels at the highest they've been for a long time.

I know this isn't sustainable for everyone and in truth I don't know how long it will be for me (I'm enjoying feeling good while it lasts though).

This tip isn't about going full-on plants only, don't worry, but increasing the amount of vegetables in your diet.

Load your lunch plate with lettuce, tomatoes, beetroot, and salad onions. For dinner give yourself double portions of broccoli and asparagus, mushrooms and onions. Not only will you feel full up more quickly (and avoid overeating the bad stuff), you'll get additional nutrients with almost no downside at all.

If you're not a big vegetable fan try eating more stir fries or chillies, and loading them with extra veggies - the texture and taste will be masked by the meat and spices, but you'll still get the benefits.

I used to avoid vegetables and convince myself that I was getting my daily portions through the vegetable components of the processed food I ate (I used to joke that I was getting a portion through eating Spicy Tomato crisps, but I think deep down I half believed it).

When I started adding vegetables to my meals rather than having them as limp steamed side portions it opened up a whole new world. (This doesn't mean if you leave your gherkins in your cheeseburger you're improving your diet.)

16. Beans

I first discovered the benefit of switching out grains to legumes thanks to Tim Ferris's Slow Carb Diet (from the highly recommended Four Hour Body).

Switching out rice in a chilli for extra kidney beans or losing the potatoes alongside the steak and replacing with lentils, initially felt like I was losing out, but as with vegetables, if you season them right then you don't notice the difference. In fact, if done right it makes for a more flavoursome and tasty meal time. Try cooking your lentils with some vegetable stock in the pan. Switch plain red kidney beans in a chilli for a can of mixed beans for variety.

Beans have a very low glycaemic index and as a result the energy is absorbed by your body at a very slow rate. As with some of the other diet tips in this book, hunger pangs between meals are minimised, and your blood sugar levels remain constant and smooth. If you're exercising you'll be able to tell the difference in performance an hour after a legume based meal rather than eating white rice or bread.

Not only that, legumes count as a vegetable, so you're killing two birds with one stone.

While some diets (including the Slow Carb) provide legumes as the main source of carbohydrates during non-cheat days, I'm not suggesting you do that. If you go full-on beans then adherence is likely to slip, and this all becomes just another fad diet. I'd recommend trying to go legumes when you can, but nothing more. Rather than having rice with your chilli every time, try and mix it up with the extra beans version every now and again. If you're having a fry up of eggs, beans, mushrooms and breakfast potatoes, try extra beans and no potatoes. Find what works for you, but if you dial up your bean consumption a little it will all add up with the other changes you're making and help with your goals.

As a footnote, if you were wondering, beans' reputation for gas is somewhat overstated in my experience. Constipation is what you need to watch out for (you have to really up your hydration while eating extra beans). Ah. We're back on the toilet again. Sorry.

17. Protein Shakes

I've spent so much money on protein shakes over the years that what I'm about to say is quite upsetting to my wallet -

"If you're a regular person, don't buy protein shakes!"

With a balanced diet it doesn't take much to get your required protein intake from the foods that you're eat. As discussed elsewhere in this book many of the good food sources you should consider adding to your diet are protein rich. Eggs, legumes, lean meat… the list goes on.

A normal person who is just looking to lose weight and stay in shape really doesn't need any further supplements.

Initially this confused me as I'd found that when I was buying and drinking shakes I was seeing better results on my diet. With hindsight this was probably due to the fact that after spending all that money on the powder I had an investment in the diet and was more likely to stick to it. To a certain extent then, protein shakes can help you stick to your goals, but that's a pretty expensive way of buying willpower, and you might be different and find it's not a motivating factor anyway.

Bottom line is - unless you're training to be a competitive body builder, save your money.

18. Fool Your Brain

So much about trying to eat healthy is a battle against your subconscious. The eating part is the tangible bit where the food actually hits your tongue and sends happy signals to your brain, but it's not just about that.

Years of associating the sound of opening a candy bar wrapper before letting it create a taste bud explosion in your mouth, the decor and sounds of entering a fast food joint before eating delicious, moorish crap, means that all of these sights, sounds and emotions are as much a part of the craving as the taste.

Trying to find replacements to trigger those same positive emotions is a great way to help beat any cravings. Here are two examples -

- When you're out with friends, or your kids, and a lunchtime fast food option looks likely, take a healthy wrap or sandwich from home and eat it in the open part of the food hall. You'll feel like you're eating in a burger joint thanks to the smell, noise and view, but you'll be eating something that's actually good for you. I don't know the science behind it but somehow when I sneak in a bagel filled with salad to eat in a McDonalds it actually tastes better than when I eat it at home.

- Try substituting a chocolate bar with a fruit bar. There's a great line of fruit bars called Nakd with flavours like Chocolate Mint, Chocolate Orange, Salted Caramel - and all they contain is fruit and nuts. They taste good, although not as nice as ACTUAL chocolate orange, but the process of opening the wrapper and feeling it in my hands scratches that particular itch and eliminates any desire for candy bars. There are other healthy treats out there of course, so give different brands a try and find the one you like best.

If there's something you particularly crave but want to try and cut down, think about the other sensations associated with it and try and recreate them alongside a healthy alternative. It really works.

19. Every Day is a Cheat Day

I don't like the concept of cheat days. Cheat days imply that for the rest of the week, you're punishing yourself by restricting what you can and can't eat, and that for one day (or meal) you can have what you want.

The Zero Effort Diet is all about having what you want, when you want. As long as you acknowledge to yourself when you're eating unhealthily and try and balance it elsewhere that day (by exercising more, or cutting back on something else) you'll be fine.

It's easy to build up to a cheat day and pig out and then go back to being healthy… but finding you had some junk left over that's still in the fridge. With all the starving people in the world it seems a shame to let it go to waste, right? Before you know it you've eaten the rest of it the following day.

I used to try and have a cheat day on a Saturday. I'd go out with my friends on a Friday night and would convince myself that my cheat 24 hours went from 6pm Friday to 6pm the next day. Looking back it was more of a cheat day and a half.

Don't think about cheat days or meals just eat "bad" stuff when you really need feel like it. By not giving yourself some self-imposed ban, you're less likely to rebel against yourself and go large.

Remember that the aim is to live a healthier lifestyle while enjoying life as it happens, not to trap yourself in a self-made cell restricting what you eat and making life miserable.

It's not cheating, it's living.

FITNESS

20. Joining a Gym

The good news is that if you're following many of the Diet tips then with practically no additional fitness work you'll start to feel better and see the weight start to fall off you. With a bit of extra effort though you can really turbocharge these results (and also make sure that you don't lose lean muscle as well as fat).

The first thing that many people think about when keeping fit is to join a gym, and for many people that's a brick wall they hit immediately. Choosing the right one takes time and effort, signing up to monthly fees, often with long term commitments, urgh. For a lot of people the effort to join starts and ends there.

Then, when you do join, you have to be disciplined enough to find the time to travel there and back (relatively easy for city dwellers with gyms in walking distance, not so easy for people who live further away). You have to try and make space in your schedule to go at least twice a week (otherwise what's the point?). Then there's the worst thing about going to a gym, if you're in anyway self-conscious - however fit and athletic you are, there will always be people there who are in far better shape than you.

Joining a gym is a great way of getting fit but not for everyone. Things to remember -

- The people that look better than you are on the same journey, just further ahead. Remember there are others that look at you, however out of shape you are, and wish they were at your level. We're all on a journey together, just at different points at any one moment in time.

- Spending money on a gym is a good motivator for actually going. You've invested your cash into it, and if you don't go you're flushing it down the toilet (if money is no object to you, then this may not apply). Either way, try and avoid a fitness centre that has a long term commitment, because if you're a regular person then at some point you're going to stop going and end up losing money, not weight.

- If you respond well to getting told what to do then getting a personal trainer at your gym is perfect for making sure you turn up every week and push yourself to the limits. If you're like me, then this is a non-starter. Someone barking orders at me doesn't motivate me to push myself harder, it motivates me to tell them where to go and walk out the place. You may be different, and if you are, a PT can have great results.

- If you're good at self-motivating, forget the gym and instead do a onetime investment in some cheap equipment for home. All you need is a weights bench, some dumbbells, and a kettlebell to have enough to do a full body workout. The total cost works out at probably no more than six months of gym fees, but it's yours forever (and if you don't use them, sell them on eBay and recoup half of your money)

21. Secret Weapon #4 - Start Swinging

If you have limited time and want one single exercise that will transform your body, then this is the one for you. After the first few sessions it will be hard to walk, and sitting down and standing up will feel like you've become 85 years old overnight, but if you can push through that then this routine will blast your core strength, your shoulders, chest, arms and legs in a full body workout that takes around 5-7 minutes.

Here it is -

Perform 75 kettlebell swings in one set, three times a week. That's it.

A kettlebell swing is where you hold the kettlebell with two hands between your legs while squatting, then swing it forward so you're standing upright and your arms are outstretched in front of you, then return to the starting position, pushing your butt out as you do it. Momentum and physics help with all of this (YouTube has untold videos showing you the correct form, so check one of those out before you attempt your first set).

The weight of the kettlebell isn't that important, so I'd start low and build up. You'll get many of the benefits with a very light weight as the squatting/swinging part of the movement is pretty unaffected. Heavier weights increase the arm/shoulder aspect of the work out.

To start with you may need to break your 75 swings into three sets of 25, or even six of 10 and one of 15. Then over subsequent sessions, up it to two of 50 and 25, and keep edging up until you can do 75 in one go.

It will hurt the next day for a while, but that five minutes of swinging is the most intense muscle building and fat burning exercise around.

I prefer to mix in smaller sets of kettlebell swings with a longer weights session, but for a long time this was my go-to body hack for toning up with minimum effort (it also gives friends and co-workers a laugh the next day when they watch you attempt to get up from sitting down, so everyone's a winner).

22. Fifteen Minute Weights

After years of trying different routines, some long (90-120 minutes every other day) and some short (like the kettlebell swings), I've discovered what I think is the ultimate time-efficient lazy-but-effective workout.

I do this three times a week. Sometimes I miss sessions, but it doesn't really matter if the goal is just to maintain muscle and feel toned. This workout won't make you massive and won't be as effective as routines that take three or four times as long, but for a fraction of the effort you'll be getting 80% of the results.

Each routine takes around 15 minutes. I perform each exercise without a break in between, with a two minute break between sets. I do this at home with dumbbells, kettlebells, and a weights bench.

Perform 10 reps of each exercise. By rep 8 onwards it should be a strain, and in the final set rep 10 should be feeling almost impossible. As you progress over the weeks, and it starts to feel like less effort, dial the weight up until you're finding the final rep a struggle again.

Monday - Chest and Biceps
Standing Dumbbell Curls
Incline Dumbbell Chest Press
Concentration Curls
Seated Row
Standing Arnold Curls

Wednesday - Shoulders and Triceps
Standing Dumbbell Shoulder Press
Standing Overhead Dumbbell Triceps Extension
Dumbbell Shrugs
Dips (I do these leaning on a dining table chair)
Standing Dumbbell Shoulder Extensions
Bent-over Dumbbell Rows

Friday - Core
Squats
Incline Crunch
Kettlebell Swings
Weighted Lunge

The motivation to start a session, even after a long day at work, or when tired in the morning, is assisted by the knowledge that in just fifteen minutes you'll be done. If you miss one it's easy to fit it in later in the day too, so adherence to this routine is high.

You can find videos showing the form and how-to's for all these exercises on YouTube or sites like www.bodybuilding.com- they're all super-easy to learn.

The most important thing about all the above is that if you start to feel a pain (not a twinge, but actual pain), then stop and leave it for a few days. It's easy to get carried away and push yourself too hard. If you're at a gym, then ask one of the trainers for assistance with form.

If you're at home, working out in front of a mirror helps so you can watch out for imbalances (i.e. leaning too much on one side). The mirror also helps when you start to tone up as you get to see the progress happening in front of your eyes.

I work out at home, as it makes me the fittest, most buff person in my personal gym (also the fattest and least fit, and the most average, but that's not how I like to think about it).

23. Walk This Way

I try and walk for an hour every day. I'm not too fussed about counting steps, or whether it's up a hill or not, just walking for an hour. There's no excuse not to track how much you walk these days, with Apple Health and Google Fit in all our pockets, and fitness bands so cheap they're given away in cereal packs (almost).

Walking gets your blood flowing, if it's outside gives you a healthy dose of vitamin D, if you're alone it can give you peaceful "you" time, and if you're with others you get to talk and exercise your brain.

Avoid public transport and your car if you can. If you work in an office, try and jump out for a walk at lunchtime. Walking is the easiest form of exercise you can do and you'll feel 100% better for doing it.

24. Running

Until a couple of years ago, I had never really been into running. Whenever I tried, I'd push myself too hard for the first half (running away from my house) and then have a walk of shame the entire way back. I got out of breath way too quickly, and I hated everything about it. I could feel my beer belly bouncing as I ran down the road, reminding me that I was overweight. The whole experience was bad and when I found that diet and weight training could help me reach my goals I consigned running to the "not for me" folder.

I hit a plateau in my routines though. I couldn't break through a certain weight barrier, and as a result my motivation for keeping up the healthy parts of my life faltered.

Then I heard about some friends who'd started running regularly after using an app called "Couch to 5k". I gave it a go, and within a couple of weeks I'd smashed through the plateau and pushed myself further than ever before. Within twelve months I ran the London 10k, a concept that a year earlier I would have laughed at. I couldn't run more than 1k without collapsing back then.

If you're already a keen runner, then excellent. If you're like I was I'd strongly advise to get out there and try it. Here are my key learnings going from a couch potato to a 10k runner -

- Buy some decent running shoes. They'll cost a bit of money but your feet will thank you. Also, you'll now be financially invested in making running work for you, making it more likely you'll keep it up.

- Use the Couch to 5k interval training plan. There are a number of apps on phones that use the routine - I used this one http://tinyurl.com/5krunner-zeroeffort. It starts off so slow and simple that I felt like a fraud for the first few days, as it's more walking than running. Don't jump ahead though. Go through the plan, and within a month you'll be amazed at your new found abilities.

- For the first few weeks, your glutes will hurt. I used to wake up in the night with seriously aching glutes. There's nothing you can do about it, just keep running and the muscle will develop and they won't ache again. Glutes by the way are your arse cheeks. If you've spent your life sat on them, it's a rude awakening to suddenly start using them. Work through it. Love your glutes.

- It doesn't matter how old you are. Anyone can start to run. There are people in their sixties and seventies running their first marathons so the age excuse is weak.

- If you're finding it hard just keep weighing yourself and measuring your waist. There's no greater motivation than seeing your body transform before your eyes.

- Get outside and run. Treadmills don't have the same effect as hitting the streets. You can set your own pace without a machine, you're in the fresh air (even if the weather's not great - running in the rain is my favourite), and you'll get less bored. Hit the streets!

By the way, while this may sound like a tip that takes more than fifteen minutes of effort, it doesn't have to. If you run for just ten solid minutes a few times a week you will reap the benefits.

25. Five Minute Wake-Up Work Out

If you're not running, and not doing weights, and the idea of kettlebell swings sound like torture, then there's one final cheat you can do that takes just five minutes and at least gets your body in tune for the day ahead.

Get in the routine of hitting the exercise bike for five minutes when you get out of bed. If you don't have a static bike, perform 10 press ups and 10 sit ups for three sets with a minute in between each one.

Do this before breakfast, literally make it the first thing you do when you get out of bed.

You won't see any rapid results but you will be getting your state of mind in the right place and preparing your body to hit the ground running for the rest of the day.

Try it and see. It's like having a quad shot espresso for stimulation.

Personally I prefer to run and do weights, but if I know I've been missing a lot of planned sessions then I try and replace them with the five minute wake up work out.

26. How to Take Measurements

Some people say not to get obsessed with measurements and to only weigh yourself or measure your waist every week or two. I couldn't disagree more.

I recommend weighing yourself every morning, before breakfast but after using the toilet. Get naked. Remove as much potential for inconsistencies as you can. Make a note of your weight, and then forget about it, so you can look at the bigger picture rather than worrying about one day's result (see tip #27).

The reason I weigh myself every day and not weekly is because even if I've had a crazy-healthy week and I'm feeling great, if it just so happens that I had a heavy meal the night before, or maybe my internal motions haven't happened as early as normal (sorry), then I could be carrying an extra couple of pounds compared to every other morning of the week. That could make it look like my weight loss has stalled, or even worse, gone backwards!

Checking weight every day eliminates this. It is what it is, and you'll get used to not getting too carried away whether it's a low or a high reading.

Other measurements are fine being checked once a week, mainly because they fluctuate less. Biceps, legs, chest etc. will grow and shrink at a snail's pace, and even the waist isn't as volatile as your actual weight. (You'll also instinctively know how your waist is doing thanks to how your clothes feel).

Body fat is one of the most important measurements to take, but it's hard to take at home accurately. You can do it with callipers but I track mine with bathroom scales. The reading is affected by how hydrated you are, so in theory first thing in the morning should be at least consistent.

As long as you're checking at a similar time every day you have relative data to track progress, even if the numbers themselves aren't quite right.

(Having said that, I paid £50 for a proper medical body fat measurement at a university once in a BodPod (www.bodpod.com) and the result was exactly the same as my "inaccurate" scales that morning... so maybe home measurements aren't that wrong after all)

27. Track Trends, Not Snapshots

Hopefully by now it's clear that the message of this book is to create a lifestyle that's healthier while not actually giving anything up and feeling like you're restricting or punishing yourself. As such, there should be no short term goals of losing "x" weight by "y" date as this is a change for life, not just a fad.

Looking at individual results when you take measurements then is the wrong thing to do. I care more about how I'm tracking over the month, or the year, rather than whether I've had an unhealthy week here or there.

I try and keep a spreadsheet with my various results so I can track trends rather than individual data, but unfortunately that requires remembering to update it, and spending time setting it up in the first place. (I'm good at the latter but not the former)

Thankfully there are a number of free websites that do this stuff for you. I use a site called Trend Weight (www.trendweight.com). You need to have Wi-Fi scales to use it, but there are others out there which let you enter the data by hand.

Rather than telling you your actual weight, it looks at your trends and tells you your trending weight. Often this will be lower or higher than your actual weight, but it's a more realistic snapshot of where you are than the number that your scales told you in the morning.

However you choose to do it, track your trends, not your daily results.

28. Secret Weapons #5 - Cold Temperature Therapy

This is the laziest and easiest secret weapon in this book. You can turbo charge your body's fat processing while sat on the sofa watching TV in the most sedentary pose imaginable.

All you need to do is buy or make a small ice pack, get it out the freezer a few times a week, and wedge it between the base of your neck and the couch. You will barely feel it as for some reason you don't feel cold there as much as elsewhere on your body. Keep it there for up to an hour, and that's it.

This is based on the concept that in freezing cold situations the body burns fat more quickly. It's why people climbing to mountain peaks, and trekking through the Arctic, eat fat supplements to counteract the loss that their bodies would otherwise suffer from.

You can go extreme with this if you want and have an ice bath, or stand in a cold shower for twenty minutes, but that's not really something I want to do. The ice pack on neck method? That's more up my street.

Add this secret weapon to your daily routine and for zero effort help freeze that fat away.

The Zero Effort Diet

GOING LARGE

29. Don't Beat Yourself Up

Sometimes you'll drink too much. Eat complete junk. Fall off the healthier lifestyle wagon with a bump. The thing to remember is… it doesn't matter. So what?

Whether you've had one night of hedonism, or a couple of weeks of forgetting any concept of attempting to be healthy, you can get back on it when you want. The worst thing you can do is feel bad about falling off the wagon and start comfort eating and drinking to make yourself feel better. That's a vicious circle led by guilt when there's no guilt to be had!

You're being healthier in some aspects of your life as a choice for You. If for some reason in your life you needed to live it large for a while, then that's also something you've done for You. So, in fact, you have stuck to your goal of "living life for You". You haven't let yourself down at all.

Try and reintroduce some of the tips in this book back into your life when you can, but don't give up. Never give up.

30. Plan Your Junk Food

If you know you're going out for a big night on the booze, and that you're going to miss dinner, or drink too much, then if you plan ahead you can minimise the amount of crap you're going to put in your body later.

Before you go out, stock up on the kind of food you'll crave after a few beers when you get home, or the unhealthy breakfast you're going to need the morning after, but buy the slightly healthier versions. You can still eat junk but at least it might be 10% healthier. Get leaner bacon, buy multigrain bread, or get a healthy choice processed microwave meal. Buy a salsa, rather than a cheese dip.

Basically, do your food shopping sober rather than when you have the munchies at the end of the night, in a supermarket rather than a convenience store that only sells processed, salt and sugar laden rubbish.

You can still eat what you want, but you're making your choices with a more sober mind. As long as you're not going large every night, it really won't make a long term difference to your goals and you won't feel like you're on a diet or being amazingly healthy. Ultimately, that's the most likely way you'll stick to it, leading to a longer, healthier, but importantly fun life.

Go out and enjoy yourself. Life's for living, and just as long as you keep things balanced you can do and achieve whatever you want.

RESOURCES

The Zero Effort Diet

You can find many of the products and gadgets mentioned in this book here. These are generally Amazon links, as the prices are often the best value there even with food and fitness products, but feel free to shop around! These are simply the products that I use - if you find similar for a cheaper price then let me know and I'll update the list for a future edition of this book.

Fitbit Wi-Fi Scales
US - http://tinyurl.com/fitbitscalesus
UK - http://tinyurl.com/fitbitscalesuk

Wi-Fi scales takes the hassle out of entering your results into various spreadsheets and tracking websites. These are FitBit scales and synchronise with a free FitBit account. You can then link to other apps and sites from there. Highly recommended.

Organic Cacao Powder
US - http://tinyurl.com/organiccacaous
UK - http://tinyurl.com/organiccacaouk

Chia Seeds
US - http://tinyurl.com/chiaseedsus
UK - http://tinyurl.com/chiaseedsuk

I didn't mention these earlier, but I put two tablespoons of chia seeds into my overnight oats recipe. They thicken the texture up a little, but more importantly are an excellent addition to your diet as they are high in fibre, protein and omega-3 fatty acids.

Truvia
US - http://tinyurl.com/truviaus
UK - http://tinyurl.com/truviauk
Truvia can be bought in your local supermarket, but this three pack offers better value for money if you're sold on using it as part of your diet.

Pre-Boiled Eggs
UK - http://tinyurl.com/preboiledeggs

Less smelly than freshly boiled eggs but just as tasty (I have three of these at one time, when I freshly boil eggs I tend to have two large ones instead).

Nutribullet Juicer
US - http://tinyurl.com/nutribulletus
UK - http://tinyurl.com/nutribulletuk

If you think that drinking fruit and veg is more likely for you than eating it fresh, then make sure you get a powerful blender like the Nutribullet juicer. This is strong enough to rip apart the flesh and innards so you retain more of the fibre and have less waste.

The Four Hour Body
US - http://tinyurl.com/4hrbody-us
UK - http://tinyurl.com/4hrbody-uk

Some interesting ideas in this book and jam packed with ideas and shortcuts to better health and fitness not just in your diet, but sleep, endurance sports, and even your sex life!

Kettlebells
US - http://tinyurl.com/kettlebellsus
UK - http://tinyurl.com/kettlebellsuk

Start small and work your way up. 75 swings of the lightest weight will still give you a work out!

Variable Weight Dumbbells
US - http://tinyurl.com/dumbells-selectableweightus
UK - http://tinyurl.com/dumbells-selectableweightuk

I have variable weight dumbbells that allow me to dial up to different weights as I'm ready for them. Much more compact and handy for a home set up than owning multiple sets of dumbbells.

Fixed Weight Dumbbells
US - http://tinyurl.com/dumbells-standardus
UK - http://tinyurl.com/dumbells-standarduk

A much more wallet friendly version of the selectable weight dumbbells. A good investment if you're just starting out and not sure if you're going to get the use out of them.

Weights Bench
US - http://tinyurl.com/weightbenchus
UK - http://tinyurl.com/weightbenchus

You don't need a bench, as most of the fifteen minute exercises can be done standing or on a chair. Some (like the incline chest press) require it though, and your general form will be better if you have a bench.

Running Shoes
US - http://tinyurl.com/runningshoesus
UK - http://tinyurl.com/runningshoesuk

These are my running shoes. As a non-runner, I found they were perfect in easing my feet into getting used to pounding the pavement. Definitely a good investment if you're serious about taking up jogging.

ABOUT THE AUTHOR

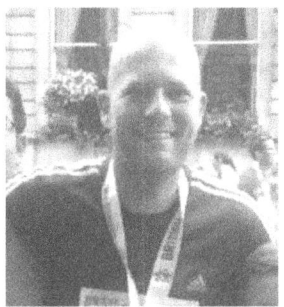

Nick Baynes is a video game director, author, serial entrepreneur and Dad, based in Brighton, UK. Join him at www.nickbaynes.com, or on Twitter @nickbaynes

Subscribe to the Zero Effort mailing list at
http://tinyurl.com/zero-effort

www.ingramcontent.com/pod-product-compliance
Lightning Source LLC
Chambersburg PA
CBHW070821290526
45795CB00002B/795